HEALING PARKINSON'S DISEASE

A COMPLETE HEALING TO PARKINSON'S DISEASE WITH CAUSES AND SYMPTOMS

DR. HYDIE BARTON

Table of Contents

CHAPTER ONE

Parkinson's disease.

Diagnosed with Parkinson's,

A degenerative brain condition, Parkinson's disease affects the parts of the brain that control movement. Slowness of movement, tremors, dizziness, and other issues are common side effects. The majority of cases are the result of random chance, but some are hereditary. Although there is no cure for this condition, there are numerous treatment options available.

Defintion of Parkinson's

When a part of your brain deteriorates, Parkinson's disease symptoms get worse over time. Muscle control, balance, and movement are the most well-known symptoms of this disorder, but it can also affect your senses, thinking, and mental health, among other things.

The average age at which Parkinson's disease begins is 60 years old, and the risk of developing it increases with age. DMAB males are slightly more likely than DMAB females to suffer from the condition, which is more common in men (DFAB).

It is not uncommon for Parkinson's disease to occur in people as young as 20 years old (though this is extremely rare, and often people have a parent, full sibling or child with the same condition).

Parkinson's disease is the second most common age-related degenerative brain disease after Alzheimer's disease. Additionally, it's the most common disease of the motor cortex in people with neurological disorders that affect movement. At least 1% of the world's population over the age of 60 is estimated to be affected.

How is this illness affecting my body??

Basal ganglia degeneration is one of the hallmarks of Parkinson's disease. In time, you will lose the abilities that you once had control over this area. Parkinson's disease has been linked to a significant alteration in the chemistry of the brain, according to recent findings.

Neurotransmitters are chemicals that your brain uses to control how your brain cells (neurons) communicate with each other under normal circumstances. Parkinson's disease is characterized by a deficiency in dopamine, a critical neurotransmitter.

Cells that need dopamine are used to fine-tune your movements when your brain sends activation signals to tell you to move. Deficiency of dopamine causes Parkinson's disease symptoms such as slowed movement and tremors.

The signs and symptoms of Parkinson's disease worsen as the condition worsens. Dementia and depression are common symptoms of Alzheimer's disease as it progresses.

When it comes to Parkinson's versus parkinsonism, what is the difference?

There are many conditions that share the symptoms of Parkinson's disease, and the term Parkinsonism is used to refer to them all. There are a variety of conditions that fall under the umbrella of "multiple system atrophy," including Parkinson's disease and corticobasal degeneration.

Causes and Symptoms

What signs and symptoms are present?

Loss of muscle control is one of the most common symptoms of Parkinson's disease. However, experts now know that Parkinson's disease isn't just a disease of the nervous system.

an issue with the motor system

Parkinson's disease has a wide range of symptoms, including the following:

• Sluggish motions (bradykinesia). This symptom is required for a diagnosis of Parkinson's disease. Those who suffer from it describe it as "muscle weakness," but in reality, there is no loss of strength.

At rest, the muscles tremble. In about 80% of Parkinson's disease cases, you'll notice a pulsating movement in your muscles even when you're not moving them. There are distinct differences between resting tremors and essential tremors.

To be rigid or stiff. Parkinson's disease is frequently accompanied by symptoms such as rigidity of lead pipes and cogwheels. This constant, unchanging stiffness is known as lead-pipe rigidity. When tremor and lead-pipe rigidity are combined, you get cogwheel stiffness. The jerky, stop-and-go movements are what give it its name (think of it as the second hand on a mechanical clock).

As a result of an unstable posture or walking gait

As Parkinson's disease progresses, a hunched or stooped posture becomes more common. This is more common as the illness progresses. Short, shuffling strides and less movement of the arms are visible when a person walks. Changing direction while walking can take several steps, depending on how far along you are.

CHAPTER TWO

Slightly fewer blinks per minute than normal. This is also a sign of facial muscle weakness.

Handwriting that is too cramped or small. It's called micrographia, and it's caused by a lack of muscle control.

• Drooling. Another symptom of facial muscle control loss is this.

Facial expression with a mask-like appearance. Facial

expressions change very little or not at all in hypomimia, a condition known as a lack of emotional expression.

• Problems with ingesting (dysphagia). When the throat muscles lose their ability to control themselves, this happens. It raises the risk of pneumonia or choking, among other things.

• Exceptionally hushed tone of voice (hypophonia). The throat and chest muscles lose their ability to control the voice.

Symptoms that are not related to the motor system

Symptoms that aren't related to movement or muscle control are possible. Non-motor symptoms were once considered risk factors for this disease by experts when they appeared before motor symptoms. Evidence suggests that these symptoms may appear even earlier in the disease's course. As a result, these symptoms could be precursors to motor symptoms that begin years or decades earlier.

In addition to the potential early warning symptoms in bold, the following non-motor symptoms may be present:

Autonomic nervous system symptoms. Constipation and other digestive and urinary issues, as well as sexual dysfunctions, are all examples of orthostatic hypotension (low blood pressure when standing).

• Depression.

Loss of smell perception (anosmia).

Periodic limb movement disorder, rapid eye movement disorder, and restless legs syndrome are all examples of sleep disorders.

Alzheimer's-related dementia can cause problems with thinking and focusing.

Parkinson's disease progression stages

Parkinson's disease can have mild symptoms for years or even decades. Margaret Hoehn and Melvin Yahr developed the Parkinson's disease staging system in 1967. It is no longer common practice to use a staging system for this condition because it is less effective than determining how it affects each person's life and then treating them accordingly.

To classify Parkinson's disease, healthcare providers use the Movement Disorder Society-Unified Parkinson's Disease Rating Scale (MDS-UPDRS). Using the MDS-UPDRS, you'll be able to see how Parkinson's disease affects you in four different ways:

There are many non-motor aspects of daily life that can be considered. Symptoms like dementia, depression, anxiety, and other mental health- and mental ability-related issues are covered in this section. Additionally, it asks questions related to pain, constipation, urinary incontinence, fatigue, and more.

• Part 2: The motor aspects of everyday experiences. • This section focuses on the effects on tasks and abilities related to movement. Speaking, eating, chewing and swallowing are all included, as are the ability to dress and bathe yourself if you have tremors.

• Motor examination in the third part. In order to determine the movement-related effects of Parkinson's disease, a healthcare provider uses this section. For example, the criteria look at things like your speech and facial expressions as well as your stiffness or rigidity in moving around, as well as how quickly you move or how fast you move.

• Complications with the motor system in the fourth part. In this section, a healthcare provider evaluates how much of a burden your Parkinson's disease symptoms are on your daily activities. The duration of symptoms and whether or not they affect how you spend your time are included in this.

What may be the cause of this?

Parkinson's disease has only one known cause: a mutation in the gene that causes Parkinson's disease. Other known risk factors for Parkinson's disease include pesticide exposure. The term "idiopathic," which means "a disease of its own" in Greek, refers to Parkinson's disease that isn't caused by a genetic mutation. This means they have no idea what causes it.

Parkinsonism (the term used to describe Parkinson's disease-like conditions caused by a specific cause, such as some psychiatric medications) is often mistaken for Parkinson's disease, but this isn't always the case.

CHAPTER THREE

Parkinson's disease in the family

Parkinson's disease can run in families, which means you may be predisposed to it if you get it from either your mother or father. However, this is the exception rather than the rule.

Parkinson's disease has been linked to at least seven different genes. Three of those have been linked to an early onset of the disease (meaning at a younger than usual age). Unique physical characteristics can also be the result of certain types of genetic mutations.

Unknown cause of Parkinson's disease

Experts believe that idiopathic Parkinson's disease is caused by a protein called -synuclein being mishandled by your body (alpha sy-nu-clee-in). When it comes to chemistry, proteins are molecules with a very specific shape. A problem known as protein misfolding prevents your body from utilizing or breaking down certain proteins.

Proteins that have nowhere else to go tend to accumulate in various locations or in specific cells (tangles or clumps of these proteins are called Lewy bodies). Toxic effects and cell damage are caused by the buildup of these Lewy bodies (which does not occur with some of the genetic problems that cause Parkinson's disease).

protein misfolding is found in a wide range of other diseases.

Parkinsonism that has been artificially induced

Experts have identified a number of factors that may contribute to the development of Parkinson's disease. In some cases, healthcare providers may consider these causes when diagnosing Parkinson's disease despite them not being true Parkinson's disease.

• Medications. Parkinsonian-like effects can be caused by several medications. If you stop taking the medication that caused the Parkinson's-like effects before they become permanent, the effects are often temporary. However, the effects of the medication can last for weeks or even months after you stop taking it.

• Encephalitis. Parkinsonism can occur as a result of encephalitis, a brain inflammation.

Toxins and poisons are substances that cause harm. Parkinsonism can be caused by a number of substances, including manganese dust, carbon monoxide fumes, welding fumes, or certain pesticides.

Injury-related damage. Repeated blows to the head, such as in sports like boxing, football, or ice hockey, can damage the brain. "Post-traumatic parkinsonism" is the medical term for this condition.

Is it spreadable?

No one else can give you Parkinson's because it is not contagious.

PHYSIOLOGY AND LAB TESTS

CHAPTER FOUR

What is the procedure for determining if this is the case?

When it comes to diagnosing Parkinson's disease, the majority of the work is done clinically, which means a doctor will ask you questions, look over your symptoms, and review your medical history. In most cases, diagnostic and laboratory tests are required to rule out other conditions or certain causes. However, unless you fail to respond to treatment for Parkinson's disease, which may indicate the presence of a different condition, most lab tests are unnecessary.

What kind of tests are going to be performed in order to determine the exact nature of this problem?

Imaging and diagnostic tests are available to rule out Parkinson's disease or other conditions when necessary. Among them are:

Testing of the blood (these can help rule out other forms of parkinsonism).

Computed tomography (CT) imaging.

Genetic testing.

• MRI, a type of X-ray imaging (MRI).

Scanning by means of positron emission tomography

There's always the possibility of additional laboratory tests.

Researchers think they've found a way to screen for the early signs of Parkinson's. There are two brand-new tests that look for the alpha-synuclein protein. In the absence of a diagnosis based on the presence of misfolded alpha-synuclein proteins, these tests can still be helpful to your doctor in establishing a diagnosis.

The following methods are used in the two tests.

• Spinal traction. Cerebrospinal fluid, the fluid that surrounds and protects your brain and spinal cord, can be tested for the presence of misfolded alpha-synuclein proteins. A healthcare provider inserts a needle into your spinal canal to collect cerebrospinal fluid for testing during a spinal tap (lumbar puncture).

biopsies of the skin. A biopsy of nerve tissue on the surface is another option. A biopsy is a procedure in which a small sample of your skin is removed and examined under a microscope. Two spots on your leg and one on your back were used to collect the samples. If your alpha-synuclein has a malfunction that could raise your risk of Parkinson's disease, analyzing the samples can help.

STRATEGIC MANAGEMENT AND MEDICATION

Is there a treatment or a cure?

Parkinson's disease cannot be cured at this time, but there are many ways to deal with the symptoms that accompany it. Additionally, the treatments can vary from person to person, depending on their specific symptoms and the effectiveness of specific treatments. This condition is primarily managed through the use of pharmaceuticals.

Implanting a mild electrical current into a portion of your brain via surgery is a second treatment option (this is known as deep brain stimulation). In addition, there are some experimental treatments, such as stem cell-based treatments, but their availability varies and many of them are not available to people with Parkinson's disease.

What types of drugs and therapies are employed?

Direct treatments and symptom treatments are the two types of Parkinson's disease medication treatments. Direct treatments focus on Parkinson's itself. Treatments for symptoms address only a subset of the disease's symptoms.

Medications

Parkinson's disease medications work in a variety of ways. Consequently, it is most likely that drugs that do the following will be used:

Dopamine can be added. It is possible to increase your brain's supply of dopamine by taking medication like levodopa. When it doesn't work, it's usually a sign of some other form of parkinsonism rather than Parkinson's disease. This medication is almost always effective. Side effects from long-term use of levodopa diminish its effectiveness.

Involved in emulating dopamine Dopamine agonists are drugs that mimic the effects of dopamine. Whenever a dopamine molecule attaches to a cell, a neurotransmitter called dopamine is released. Dopamine agonists are capable of binding to cells and causing them to behave in a similar manner.. There is a higher incidence of these in younger patients in order to delay the onset of levodopa therapy.

Blockers of the dopamine metabolism. Dopamine is a neurotransmitter that is naturally broken down by your body. More dopamine is available to the brain when your body is prevented from breaking down the chemical. They're particularly helpful in the early stages of Parkinson's disease, but they can also be helpful in conjunction with levodopa in later stages.

Inhibitors of the metabolism of levodopa Levodopa lasts longer when your body slows down the rate at which it is metabolized by these medications. Toxic effects and liver damage are possible with these medications, so use with caution. The most common reason for using them is when levodopa becomes ineffective.

Blockers of the adenosine receptor. When taken with levodopa, medications that interfere with the way certain cells use adenosine (a molecule found in many different forms throughout your body) may be helpful.

Parkinson's disease-specific symptoms are addressed by a variety of medications. The following are some of the most common conditions that are treated:

CHAPTER FIVE

Sexual and erection problems.

- Tiredness or drowsiness.

- Constipation.

Problems with sleep.

- Depression.

- Dementia.

- Anxiety.

- Psychotic symptoms such as hallucinations and delusions.

Stimulation of the deep brain

When it comes to treating Parkinson's disease, surgery was once an option that allowed you to intentionally damage and scar a part of your brain that was malfunctioning. Deep-brain stimulation, which uses an implanted device to deliver a mild electrical current to those same areas, can now achieve the same result.

Because deep-brain stimulation is reversible, it has a major advantage over intentional scarring. For people with Parkinson's disease who have tremors that don't seem to respond to the usual medications, this treatment approach is almost always an option.

Treatments that have not yet been proven effective.

Parkinson's disease researchers are looking into other possible treatments. They may not be widely available, but they offer some hope to those who suffer from this disease. Treatment approaches that are currently being tested include the following:

Transplantation of stem cells Your brain is given new dopamine-producing neurons to replace those that have died.

The treatment of damaged neurons. These therapies aim to repair and regenerate neurons, as well as to stimulate the growth of new ones.

• Gene therapies and treatments that target specific genes. There are specific mutations in the brain that cause Parkinson's disease, and these treatments aim to correct those problems. Levodopa and other treatments can benefit from some of these supplements as well.

Treatments may cause complications or side effects.

Parkinson's disease treatment complications and side effects are influenced by a variety of factors, including the type of treatment used, the severity of the disease, and any other health issues you may be dealing with. When it comes to potential side effects and complications, your healthcare provider is your best source of information. They can also give you advice on how to lessen the impact of any negative effects or complications.

Learn about levodopa.

For Parkinson's disease, levodopa is by far the most common and best-known drug therapy. However, because of the way it works, doctors are cautious when prescribing this medication for Parkinson's patients. Levodopa is frequently combined with other drugs to increase its effectiveness or alleviate its side effects and symptoms.

Because your body can't process levodopa before it enters your brain, you often take it with other drugs. Dopamine side effects such as nausea, vomiting, and a drop in blood pressure when you stand up can be avoided in this way (orthostatic hypotension).

Levodopa's effectiveness diminishes over time as your body adapts to the drug. There is a chance that increasing your dosage will help, but it will also increase your risk of side effects, and the dose can only go so high before it's toxic level.

What can I do to better take care of myself and lessen the effects of these symptoms?

No one should attempt to self-diagnose Parkinson's disease or treat its symptoms without first consulting a medical professional.

How quickly will I begin to feel better, and how long will it take for my body to return to normal?

How quickly a person with Parkinson's disease recovers and experiences the benefits of treatment varies greatly depending on the type of treatment used and how severe their condition is. The best source of information on what to expect from treatment is your doctor or other medical professional. The data they provide can take into account any particulars specific to your situation.

CHAPTER SIX

What can I do to lessen or eliminate my exposure to this ailment?

Parkinson's disease can be caused by a combination of genetic and environmental factors. Both are not preventable, and you cannot lower your risk of developing it. Not everyone who works in farming or welding is at risk for developing Parkinson's disease.

The prognosis or outlook

As a result, what should I be prepared for?

PD is a degenerative disease, which means that its effects on the brain worsen over time. However, the deterioration of this condition typically takes a long time. People with this condition typically live healthy, normal lives.

Early on, you won't require much assistance and can continue to live on your own. There are medications that can help alleviate the symptoms as they worsen. As soon as your doctor determines the lowest effective dose of most medications, such as levodopa, it can be moderately or even very effective in treating your symptoms.

As time goes on, treatment options become less effective and more difficult to manage for many of the symptoms. As the disease progresses, it will become increasingly difficult to live on one's own.

Does Parkinson's disease last forever?

Parkinson's disease is incurable, so it will affect you for the rest of your life.

What is the prognosis of Parkinson's?

Parkinson's disease does not cause death, but its symptoms and consequences often do. It was estimated that Parkinson's disease patients had a 10-year lifespan in 1967. Average life expectancy has increased by 55% since then, reaching more than 14.5 years Because

Parkinson's diagnosis is more common after the age of 60, it doesn't usually affect your life expectancy by more than a few years (depending on the life expectancy in your country).

SHARING A HOME WITH OTHERS

How do I take care of my own needs?

The best thing you can do if you have Parkinson's disease is to follow the advice of your healthcare provider.

• Follow the directions on the label of the medication you are taking. You can make a huge difference in the symptoms of Parkinson's disease by taking your medication. When taking medication, follow the directions on the label and consult your doctor if you experience any side effects or begin to question the efficacy of your prescriptions.

• Follow the advice of your healthcare professional and make an appointment with them. You will have an appointment with your healthcare provider on a specific day and time. These appointments are critical for keeping your health under control and determining the best medications and dosages for you.

• Don't ignore or avoid the symptoms of a disease. Several symptoms of Parkinson's disease can be treated by addressing the underlying cause of the disease or addressing the symptoms directly. Treatment can prevent symptoms from worsening significantly.

What is the best time to see a doctor or get medical attention?

If your symptoms or medication effectiveness change, or if your healthcare provider recommends it, you should make an appointment with them. Parkinson's disease can be greatly improved by making minor adjustments to medication and dosage.

When should I go to the emergency room?

You can get advice and information from your

healthcare provider about signs and symptoms that indicate that you need to go to the hospital or get medical attention. In general, if you fall and lose consciousness or suffer an injury to your head, neck, chest, back, or abdomen, you should seek medical attention.

Inquiries that are frequently requested

Parkinson's disease develops for unknown reasons.

It is not known why the vast majority of Parkinson's disease cases occur. Approximately 10% of cases are inherited, which means that one or both of your parents have them. However, the remaining 90 percent or so are idiopathic, which means they occur for unknown reasons.

Parkinson's disease has early warning signs, but what are they?

Slowness of movement, tremors, or stiffness are some of the motor symptoms that may indicate Parkinson's disease. Non-motor symptoms, on the other hand, are possible. There are a number of non-motor symptoms that may begin to appear years or even decades before motor symptoms. Non-motor symptoms, on the other hand, can be difficult to link to Parkinson's disease because they can be so vague.

There are a number of non-motor symptoms that could serve as early warning signs.

Autonomic nervous system symptoms. Constipation and lightheadedness upon standing are among the symptoms of orthostatic hypotension.

Loss of smell perception (anosmia).

Periodic limb movement disorder, rapid eye movement disorder, and restless legs syndrome are all examples of sleep disorders.

How long does it take to die from Parkinson's?

Parkinson's disease itself does not cause death. It can, however, cause other, potentially fatal conditions or problems.

Sadly, Parkinson's disease cannot be cured. There are many effective treatments for this condition, however. Another possibility is to slow down the disease's progression.

Cleveland Clinic issued a statement

As people age, they are more likely to develop Parkinson's disease, which is a common condition. Although Parkinson's is not reversible, there are numerous treatment options available to those with the disease. They include a variety of medications, surgery to implant brain-stimulating devices, and other treatments. Advances in treatment and care have made it possible for many people with this condition to live for many years or even decades.

THE END